T0148450

DIABETES:
Can It Be Reversed?

DIABETES:
Can It Be Reversed?

What Your Doctor May Not Want to Tell You!

Dr. E. Barrett Hall

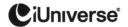

DIABETES: CAN IT BE REVERSED?
WHAT YOUR DOCTOR MAY NOT WANT TO TELL YOU!

iUniverse books may be ordered through booksellers or by contacting:

iUniverse
1663 Liberty Drive
Bloomington, IN 47403
www.iuniverse.com
1-800-Authors (1-800-288-4677)

ISBN: 978-1-4917-6387-2 (sc)
ISBN: 978-1-4917-6386-5 (e)

Library of Congress Control Number: 2015906651

Print information available on the last page.

iUniverse rev. date: 06/26/2015

Contents

Disclaimer

Although the author and publisher have made every effort to ensure that the information in this book was correct at press time, the author and publisher do not assume and hereby disclaim any liability to any party for any loss, damage, or disruption caused by errors or omissions, whether such errors or omissions result from negligence, accident, or any other cause.

The material in this book is intended to provide information on a disease (diabetes) that has become a scourge, reaching epidemic proportions in the United States and the rest of the world. The information shared in this book is based upon research and personal experience. The information is presented for information purposes only and is not intended to replace treatment received from your medical practitioner.

The reader should regularly consult a physician (doctor) in matters relating to his or her health, particularly with respect to any symptoms that may require diagnosis or immediate medical attention. If you desire to take supplements or make dietary changes, please consult your doctor before doing so. If your doctor prescribed medication, please follow his or her instructions. You should not stop taking your prescribed medication without your doctor's permission.

Preface

Why this book? Hello, my name is Dr. Esric Hall. In 2009 I was diagnosed with type 2 diabetes. Before I go any further, I must stress that I am not a medical doctor. I have a doctorate degree from a prestigious university and have used my research capabilities to study diabetes, especially type 2 diabetes. Since my diagnosis, it has been a struggle to get my blood sugar under control. During one of my visits to my primary care physician, I was told I might be put on insulin if I was unable to get my blood sugar under control with oral medication. In all honesty, there is nothing wrong with giving yourself insulin shots. Insulin is pure and is probably one of the better treatments available for this disease, but I did not want to give myself daily injections.

I recently focused my research on the source of the problem, trying to understand it from the molecular level. I wanted to know what had gone wrong in my body that had resulted in this disease. What I have uncovered is astounding. I am convinced this is a disease that can be reversed. From my research, it appears that most doctors do not truly understand diabetes and how to treat it. In this book, I provide some easy-to-follow steps that have helped keep my blood glucose level under control. Because of what I uncovered and its implications for other people with this disease, I felt obliged to share this information, and what better forum to do so than in a book!

CHAPTER 1

Diabetes Introduced

D iabetes: What is it? Diabetes, also referred to as *diabetes mellitus*, is a metabolic disease (although some classify it as autoimmune) in which the body does not use glucose effectively, resulting in high blood sugar in the bloodstream. *Metabolic disease* simply means your body is unable to break down food properly so that it can be converted into energy. *Autoimmune disease*, on the other hand, refers to something that has gone wrong in your immune system, causing an overreaction by your body; in the case of diabetes, this affects insulin production. Diabetes may be classified into four types, including prediabetes. These are introduced here but discussed further in chapter 2.

Prediabetes: Before someone develops type 2 diabetes, he or she usually has prediabetes, in which blood glucose levels are elevated but are not high enough for the patient to be classified as having type 2.

Type 1: The body no longer produces insulin (the hormone

responsible for transporting the sugar from the bloodstream to the cells).

Type 2: The body still makes insulin but fails to use it effectively. This is also known as non–insulin dependent diabetes.

Gestational: This occurs during pregnancy—usually around the twenty fourth week—due to hormonal changes. This does not mean that the expectant mother will develop full-blown diabetes, but following doctor's orders is of utmost importance.

Prevalence: Diabetes has now reached epidemic proportions in the United States and around the world. There are approximately 350 million cases worldwide, and in the United States alone— according to data from the Center for Disease Control *National Diabetes Statistics* report of 2014—the total prevalence is 29.1 million children and adults, which represents 9.3 percent of the population. Of the 29.1 million cases, it is believed that 21 million people have been diagnosed, and the remaining 8.9 million people are still undiagnosed. Prediabetics alone number 79 million people. (http://www.cdc.gov/diabetes/data/statistics/2014StatisticsReport.html)

New Cases: 1.9 million new cases of diabetes were diagnosed in people aged twenty years and older in 2010. Based on this statistic, it is safe to say we are approaching epidemic proportions for this disease worldwide. Current projections put half of the US population at risk for type 2 diabetes by the year 2020, a figure that would represent a 98 percent rise. Many years ago, type 2 diabetes was mainly a disease that adults contracted. Nowadays, kids are contracting type 2 diabetes at an alarming rate (http://www.diabetes.org/diabetes-basics/statistics/). According to an ABC news article November 2010, it is projected that that if current trends continue, half of the American adults are headed for diabetes by 2020 (http://abcnews.go.com/Health/Diabetes/diabetes-half-us-adults-risk-2020-unitedhealth-group/story?id=12238602).

For approximately two weeks before I was diagnosed with diabetes, I observed distinct changes in the way my face looked; to put it frankly, I looked like hell. I also had a persistent thirst. I was going through at least a couple of two-liter bottles of cranberry juice daily, which at that time was my beverage of choice. I had no idea what was going on. I would also wake up in the middle of the night a few times to urinate. I also noticed that I was losing a lot of weight, but I attributed that to biking, which I did every day. At work I had started to get double takes from people who knew me—*and* from folks who did not know me; that was a good indication that I looked like hell. I also fielded questions as to whether or not I was on a diet. I looked pretty bad, and I had no idea what was going on.

My next move, of course, was to go to the doctor. Prior to my doctor's visit I researched my symptoms on the Internet and got the shocker that it may be diabetes. My first reaction was *this is impossible … this disease happens to other people.* No one in my family had ever had diabetes, and I understood this disease was hereditary. In a nutshell, my thinking was that diabetes was someone else's concern, not mine. I was in for a big surprise. My doctor confirmed that I had type 2 diabetes. My blood sugar was 427 mg/dL, meaning there were 427 milligrams of sugar for every deciliter (one tenth of a liter) of blood. At the time I did not understand what that number meant, but when I learned more about the disease, you can just imagine I was shocked. Anyway, I survived and started on the journey of prescription medication.

Prior to being diagnosed with type 2 diabetes, I had been fairly healthy. I often had bouts with allergies, but that had been the extent of my illnesses. Now I was entering into a strange and seemingly dark world of despair. The thought of losing my sight and limbs and eventually succumbing to complications caused by this disease put tremendous fear in me.

After my diagnosis, my life changed. I could not eat my favorite snack (ice cream), and I had to follow a special diet and count carbohydrates (carbs). For those of you who are not aware, counting carbs involves reading food labels and then trying to balance meals to reduce carbohydrate intake. If you have not heard the term before, carbohydrates are sugars and starches. All the food we eat eventually gets converted into energy for use by our bodies. Some foods are high in carbohydrates, some are high in protein, and others are high in fat. These are the three main energy sources we receive from the food we eat. In addition to counting carbs, you also learn how many grams of carbohydrates are in each serving of foods such as rice, french fries, and other similar foods. It is therefore extremely important to know how to count carbohydrate content to keep carbohydrate intake to a minimum. Why do we want to pay special attention to carbs? Because foods rich in carbohydrates are almost instantly converted to sugar after they are consumed—not good news if you have diabetes.

I thought for sure that getting diabetes was punishment for a lifetime of not paying attention to my diet. I started doing research on the disease to find which supplements would help me control my diabetes; I wanted to know what I could take to allow the glucose to move into the cells in my body in a timely manner. Based on the results of this first research, I added chromium, vanadium, and cinnamon to the multivitamins I had been taking for many years. During the first year, I must admit I did an excellent job managing the disease. I biked daily when the weather permitted, I was very careful about what I ate, and I reduced my carbohydrate intake significantly. Of course I was still skinny and I was half starving myself, but my face did not have that sickly look as it had before. I no longer got double takes.

My first doctor's visit after my diagnosis revealed that my A1c levels had gone down from a little over 12 percent (extremely dangerous) to approximately 8 percent (still not ideal). The hemoglobin A1c (HbA1c) blood test is a tool used in the management of diabetes.

HbA1c measures the glucose levels in the bloodstream over a period of generally six to twelve weeks. The hemoglobin A1c level for a healthy adult is usually less than 5.9 percent. The recommended treatment goals for diabetic adults for hemoglobin A1c are to achieve levels below 7 percent. So how does A1c work? A1c measures an average of your blood glucose level twenty-four hours per day. Hemoglobin, a protein in the red blood cells, links up (glycates) with the sugar in the blood. As these cells move through, some glucose (sugar) in the bloodstream becomes attached to these cells. The more sugar there is in the blood stream, the higher the percentage of A1c cells that will have glucose attached. The lifespan of A1c cells is approximately four months, and measuring the level of A1c in the blood cells over a three-month period is one of the most popular and accurate methods used to measure blood sugar control.

After my second doctor's visit, my A1c level was under 7 percent. I was in control. I must warn you, however: if you are a newly diagnosed diabetic or prediabetic, be very careful. It is easy to become complacent thinking that you have licked this disease, and that is understandable. If your blood sugar readings are normal and you are feeling healthy, don't forget that your body is still out of whack. There is a reason you have diabetes; something in your body is not functioning properly, and until you are able to understand the problem and take steps to remedy the condition, you will have limited success. You have organs that have become tired or sick and need time to heal. These concepts of giving your body time to heal and build strength to attack the disease at the source (molecular level) are the underlying principles of this book.

Diabetes is a disease that can and will get progressively worse, especially if it is not adequately managed. To effectively manage diabetes, one requires major lifestyle changes, including healthy eating habits, stress management, and exercise. Learning how to manage diabetes has been by far one of the biggest struggles of my entire life. During the second year after my diagnosis, my life changed somewhat. I moved into a different house, and some of the amenities I had become accustomed to were no longer available. There were no bike tracks close by (I am an avid bike rider), and I did not make the effort to join a gym. Consequently, my blood sugar stayed in the high range due to a somewhat sedentary lifestyle. My main activity after work was watching television. The lack of exercise and my new TV habit were a recipe for disaster.

Various studies—too many to list here—have shown that regular exercise can significantly reduce blood glucose levels. A word of warning about exercise, however: moderate exercise is recommended, as is weight training to strengthen muscles. However, exercise that is too rigorous may cause your body to view the event as stressful, and it may release excess sugar and consequently raise blood sugar levels. Due to my inactivity, life stressors, and a bit of complacency (not paying close attention to what I was eating), my blood sugar control was not as good as it had been during my first year. My doctor indicated I may need to be put on insulin, and that is when I went to work. Insulin therapy is probably one of the better treatments for diabetes. When injected, it takes over the insulin function of the pancreas, which is now producing less insulin or in some cases—as in type 1 diabetes—no insulin. Although insulin is a proven treatment, I did not care to give myself injections.

In order to manage diabetes and reverse it, one must understand the cause and then attack it at its source. After reading this chapter, you should have a better understanding of the nuances or—to put it in simpler terms—the strange twists of diabetes. You will learn about foods to avoid and learn of new and promising research and treatments. You will determine whether your current treatment path for this disease is adequate, and if it is not you'll learn how to make the required changes. You will also be able understand the disease from the molecular level, and why treatment from this perspective makes sense.

CHAPTER 2

Diabetes Explored

So why is insulin important? When you eat, food is converted to glucose, the fuel that keeps cells alive and well. One of the functions of insulin is to transport the glucose into the cells in your body. When the body stops producing insulin or cannot recognize and use it efficiently, then diabetes sets in.

What do we mean by *insulin resistance* or *insulin depletion*? In the pancreas there are specialized hormone-producing cells known as *beta cells*. These cells produce insulin, which helps regulate blood sugar. A single beta cell can make a million molecules of insulin a minute. If these beta cells are damaged or destroyed, then insulin production is affected or completely lost.

When the pancreas cannot produce sufficient insulin—or, in the case of type 1 diabetes, does not produce any—the cells in our bodies become starved of fuel (glucose). Sugar remains in the bloodstream and is subsequently passed in the urine. This explains the frequent urination as one of the symptoms of high blood sugar; most of the nutrients the body needs for sustainment are passed in the urine, resulting in significant weight loss. This usually happens at the onset of the disease or when the disease is not properly managed and blood sugar levels are elevated.

Prior to being diagnosed with diabetes, I weighed approximately 190 lbs. I did not have a potbelly, which is closely associated with developing type 2 diabetes. I exercised regularly, so in my case it is clear that obesity was not the cause. Current research shows that the leading cause of diabetes is inflammation of the pancreas. This inflammation is hidden and can start a long time before you know you have diabetes. When the pancreas gets damaged, it cannot meet the insulin requirements of the body.

In a healthy person the pancreas releases insulin, which moves the glucose from the bloodstream into the cells to help the body store and use sugar. Diabetes can occur when the pancreas has stopped producing insulin (type 1 diabetes), when the pancreas does not produce sufficient insulin, or when the body simply does not utilize the insulin properly (type 2 diabetes).

- **PREDIABETES**

In prediabetes, blood sugar is sometimes above the normal range of 70 to 100 milligrams per deciliter. This is often referred to as *impaired glucose tolerance* and the blood sugar level is not high enough to be classified as type 2 diabetes. Blood sugar level testing should be done after fasting (six to eight hours after the last meal). To check for diabetes, this is generally done first thing in the morning before having breakfast. During the day, random glucose testing can be done to give an idea of the range of blood sugar levels during the day. You may also elect to do testing two hours after a meal (two-hour postprandial blood sugar), another method used to diagnose diabetes. When you have a meal, blood sugar generally rises, and in a normal individual it usually does not get above 135 to 140 milligrams per deciliter. So there is a fairly narrow range of blood sugar levels throughout the day.

- ## TYPE 2 DIABETES

Type 2 diabetes, also known as *non–insulin dependent diabetes mellitus* (NIDDM), is the most common form of diabetes. Millions have been diagnosed with type 2 diabetes in the United States, and millions more are at risk. In type 2 diabetes, the body still produces insulin but it is not used efficiently (insulin resistant). When we eat, the body breaks down food into glucose, which is then transported into the cells by insulin. When the body does not recognize the presence of insulin, too much sugar builds up in the bloodstream and it is not transported into the cells. This is also similar to what happens in gestational diabetes, to which pregnant women are susceptible. In chapter 1, I indicated that diabetes is considered a metabolic disorder; a recent study published in *Nature Medicine* mentions that type 2 diabetes is in the process of being redefined as an autoimmune disorder (http://www.medicalnewstoday.com/articles/222766.php).

- ## GESTATIONAL DIABETES

Gestational diabetes can befall women in several stages of pregnancy. This is also a condition similar to type 2 diabetes in which the body shows intolerance to glucose and is not able to use all of the insulin needed because the insulin receptors have malfunctioned. This condition generally has few symptoms and is usually diagnosed during screening. If left unmanaged, however, gestational diabetes can develop into type 2 diabetes and, in rare cases, type 1. It is unknown why pregnant women develop diabetes, but one contributing factor is that certain hormones that are required for a baby's development can block insulin.

• TYPE 1 DIABETES

Type 1 diabetes—also called *juvenile diabetes* or *insulin dependent diabetes mellitus* (IDDM)—is usually diagnosed in young adults and children. The onset of type 1 is usually fast and furious; consequently, it is usually diagnosed in a hospital emergency room. In type 1 diabetes, the body does not produce insulin. The beta cells in the pancreas, which are responsible for insulin production, may be completely destroyed. Type 1 diabetes treatment requires multiple daily injections of insulin. Insulin is the hormone produced by the beta cells in the pancreas and its purpose is to transport the sugar from the bloodstream into the cells. When you eat, food is converted into fuel in the form of glucose, and the cells need this glucose for energy. People with type 1 diabetes must take insulin injections.

What Is the Cause of Diabetes?

There are many theories on what causes diabetes. It has often been written that obesity, poor diet, and lack of physical exercise are leading causes. It has also been written that a sedentary lifestyle is another culprit. People who are obese may have a greater susceptibility to the disease. There is more sugar in your system if you are obese, and this excess may be taxing your digestive system, which includes insulin production and blood glucose removal from the bloodstream. Research shows that there are a number of contributing factors linked to developing diabetes, and chief among them is metabolic syndrome X.

- **METABOLIC SYNDROME X**

This factor represents a collection of medical disorders which when they occur together increases the risk of cardiovascular disease and diabetes. When describing metabolic syndrome X, there are varying guidelines from many organizations that dictate whether or not one is suffering from this condition, including the World Health Organization (WHO), the American Heart Association, the International Diabetes Federation (IDF), and the National Cholesterol Education Program (NCEP). The consensus is that if you are overweight and have two or more of the following, you are at risk for syndrome X:

- ✓ raised triglycerides > 150 mg/dL

- ✓ reduced HDL cholesterol < 40 mg/dL in males and < 50 mg /dL in females

- ✓ raised fasting glucose > 100 mg/dL

✓ Raised blood pressure systolic BP > 130 mm Hg or diastolic > 85 mm Hg

Please note these numbers vary slightly from one organization to the next. Studies have shown that, in addition to these risk factors, poor diet and stress can also be contributing factors (http://www.diabetes. org/living-with-diabetes/complications/mental-health/stress.html, http://www.webmd.com/diabetes/features/stress-diabetes).

- **POOR DIET**

Poor diet has been shown to contribute to developing diabetes, especially type 2 (http://www.livestrong.com/article/445709-can-a-poor-diet-cause-diabetes/). Eating healthy is not only important in the prevention of diabetes, but also it is essential for those of us who already have the disease. By following a proper diet, you set the stage for a healthier lifestyle and lay the groundwork necessary for reversing this debilitating disease. Diets high in fat, such as fried foods high in hydrogenated trans-fatty-acids, should be avoided. For frying, choose your oil carefully. Coconut or peanut oils are safe choices; these oils do not break down when heated. Other oils may break down upon heating and create free radicals. Stay away from food high in sugar and also processed food; these are poor choices. Other issues that can result from poor diet are mineral deficiencies, food toxins that create free radicals, and insufficient digestion. Eat whole grains, fruits, vegetables, protein, and healthy fats, such as polyunsaturated and monounsaturated fats; also limit consuming food high in sugar.

In this section I will cover two food additives that you should avoid. If you are not in the habit of reading food labels, I suggest this is a good time to start; it could save your life.

✓ *High fructose corn syrup*: Studies have shown that this food additive could contribute to developing diabetes. The study published in the journal *Global Health* found an association between diabetes and high fructose corn syrup, but did not establish that high fructose corn syrup *caused* diabetes. However, the results show that countries that use high fructose corn syrup had a diabetes rate twenty times greater than countries that did not use it. (http://www. ncbi.nlm.nih.gov/pubmed/23181629.) This additive is in almost everything we eat, including bread, fruit juices, ketchup, cereal, and soda. This is a cheap additive that may be harming us; it causes increased uric acid levels in your body and produces new fat cells around vital organs such as the liver, heart, and other digestive organs. As mentioned before, I recommend reading the labels on food products and making informed decisions.

✓ *Aspartame*: This is frequently referred to as one of the most dangerous food additives on the market, and consumption can lead to serious health problems. Reported symptoms of aspartame include: headaches, memory loss, joint pain, anxiety attacks, slurred speech, heart palpitations, breathing problems, muscle spasms, nausea, numbness, convulsions, weight gain, rashes, depression, fatigue, irritability, vision problems, and hearing problems. These are just a few of the ninety documented symptoms reported to the Food and Drug Administration (FDA) by the Aspartame Toxicity Information Center and available at the FDA.gov website http://www.fda.gov/RegulatoryInformation/Dockets/ default.htm). In addition, some chronic diseases can be worsened if aspartame is ingested. These include diabetes, fibromyalgia, birth defects, lymphoma, mental retardation, Alzheimer's disease, Parkinson's disease, brain tumors, multiple sclerosis, epilepsy, and chronic fatigue syndrome. This sweetener is found in some low-calorie sweeteners and diet sodas.

People with diabetes looking for a better alternative may use products containing aspartame. Again, please read the food labels and choose your food wisely. There is some concern that aspartame may be linked to brain tumors. A study conducted at Washington University Medical School show some connection between rats that were fed aspartame and increased brain tumors.

- **STRESS**

Stress control is important in managing diabetes. A study conducted by researchers at the University of Gothenburg in Sweden showed that men who were permanently stressed significantly increased the risk of developing type 2 diabetes. Stress can be in the form of physical stress or mental stress; it causes the body to act as if it is under attack, thus creating the *fight-or-flight syndrome*. Physical stress occurs when the body is recuperating from something physical such as surgery or injury. Mental stress causes the body to go into that fight-or-flight mode, and in preparing for this, hormone levels in the body rise, releasing stored energy (glucose) to the cells to help the body deal with this perceived danger. In people with diabetes especially type 2 this extra glucose is not absorbed in the body cells, and it piles up in the bloodstream; the end result is high blood sugar. So whether you have diabetes or not, stress can be very harmful to your health. Therefore it is very important that you seek out and find ways to reduce stress (http://www.webmd.com/diabetes/features/stress–diabetes).

- **VITAMIN D DEFICIENCY**

Recent studies have shown that vitamin D deficiency may contribute to developing both type 1 and type 2 diabetes in both humans and animals, as it has been found to impair insulin function. We typically get vitamin D from exposure to sunlight and also from naturally occurring sources in foods such as eggs, cod, and salmon. People with darker complexions may not get sufficient vitamin D due to the higher level of the pigment melanin in the skin, since melanin blocks the nutrient from being absorbed in the body. Vitamin D has also been shown to help prevent at-risk individuals from developing diabetes. (http://www.naturalnews. com/028355_vitamin_D_insulin_sensitivity.html), http://ajcn. nutrition.org/content/79/3/362.short, http://link.springer.com/ article/10.1007/s00125-004-1329-3#page-1, http://europepmc.org/ abstract/med/12800453.

* **AGE**

As we age, so does every organ in our bodies. Our ability to digest sugar also slows down. This is one reason that the onslaught of type 2 diabetes afflicts mostly adults; this is a time when the body is wearing out and more likely to have insulin resistance. From the cellular level, as we get older the beta cells in the pancreas responsible for producing insulin get tired and worn down. At this stage of the game there are also far fewer of them. Good diet is important: limit the intake of sugar and complex carbohydrates, which take a long time to digest and can result in hyperglycemia. (http://www.ncbi. nlm.nih.gov/pmc/articles/PMC3164365/).

* **B CELLS ATTACK BODY TISSUE**

Type 2 diabetes is in the process of being redefined as an autoimmune disorder. Recent studies have shown that the B cells in the immune system, which are mostly responsible for antibody responses, can cause inflammation and lead to developing diabetes. In a study published in *Nature Medicine*, mice were genetically engineered to lack B cells. These mice were then fed a high-fat, high-calorie diet, and they did not develop diabetes. The mice were then injected with B cells from obese mice that were insulin resistant; the mice then developed insulin resistance. Although this result was found in mice,

B cells in humans have the same function to protect the body from infection, although these cells also have the ability to cause disease. (http://www.medicalnewstoday.com/articles/222766.php).

- ## DIABETES CONNECTION TO PH BALANCE

People with diabetes encounter dehydration problems; fluids are expelled as soon as they go in. The body is fighting to maintain a pH balance that is too acidic, but it is difficult to maintain a more alkaline environment because the cells cannot sufficiently absorb the proper amount of nutrients. Before I continue, let's discuss pH balance. What is it?

A pH number is measured on a scale from 0 to 14. This number tells how acidic or alkaline something is. Any number above 7 is considered alkaline, and any number below 7 is considered acidic. Water, for example, has a pH level of 7, meaning it has the same amount of acids and alkalis, which balance each other out. For good health, we aim to have acidic levels of 7.3 to 7.45, meaning our bodies should be slightly acidic but very close to neutral (http://www.mindbodygreen.com/0-6243/How-to-Balance-Your-pH-to-Heal-Your-Body.html). When the cells don't work properly, neither do the organs; therefore, if you are diabetic, chances are you already have a pH balance that is too acidic. If you don't reduce the acid in your body, you could end up developing complications such as kidney failure, gangrene, and blindness.

Blood sugar balance is critical to your body's proper functioning. Blood sugar is the primary source of fuel for the body's cells and is particularly critical to the brain and eyes. When glucose isn't regulated properly through the bloodstream, the body's cells don't get the energy they need. When you have excessively high blood sugar (hyperglycemia) or excessively low blood sugar (hypoglycemia), it prevents the organs from working properly and leads to a decline in health and faster aging process.

The body's blood sugar level is regulated primarily by the pancreas and liver. The liver stores excess glucose and releases it when needed. The pancreas secretes insulin that helps carry glucose into the body's cells, and it secretes glucagon that triggers the release of stored glucose in the liver. When the body becomes too acidic, it can affect either organ from functioning properly, causing the blood sugar to become excessively high or low. Unless this process is reversed, the cells will begin to starve.

Having a highly acidic pH balance level can put the pancreas, liver, and all the body's organs at risk. Because of the important role played by the liver in removing acid waste from the body, liver function is particularly at risk when acids accumulate.

Traditional medicines derived from medicinal plants are used by about 60 percent of the world's population. This review focuses on Indian herbal drugs and plants used in the treatment of diabetes, especially in India. Diabetes is an important human ailment afflicting many from various walks of life in different countries. In India, it is proving to be a major health problem, especially in urban areas. According to an article in *Time*, there are no good answers for the diabetes crisis that India currently faces (http://world.time.com/2013/05/12/no-answers-in-sight-for-indias-diabetes-crisis/). Although there are various approaches to reduce the ill effects of diabetes and its secondary complications, herbal formulations are preferred due to fewer side effects and lower cost.

A list of medicinal plants with proven antidiabetic and related beneficial effects and of herbal drugs used in treatment of diabetes is provided in chapter 7.

One of the etiologic (risk) factors implicated in the development of diabetes and its complications is the damage induced by oxidative stress; hence an antidiabetic compound with antioxidant properties would be more beneficial. For this reason, information on antioxidant effects of these medicinal plants is also included.

• OXIDATIVE STRESS

One report indicates the following: researchers are in basic agreement that the theory of oxidative stress is essential to explaining one of the causes of diabetes. To understand the theory, one must first conceptualize that a *free radical* is any atom or molecule that has an unpaired electron in its outer ring. Because it is lacking an electron, it is unstable and very much wants to find one electron to fill its need. This free radical will steal an electron from any other molecule it encounters that is more willing to give one up; thus it becomes satisfied. The victim molecule now becomes a free radical itself, however, and will look for another victim molecule to steal its much desired electron from—thus propagating the cycle over and over again. This cycle is called *the chain reaction of free radicals* (http://diabetesherbal.com/oxidativestress.php).

The chief danger of free radicals comes from the damage they can do when they react with important cellular components such as DNA (deoxyribonucleic acid), the hereditary material in humans and almost all other organisms, or the cell membrane. Cells may function poorly or die if this occurs.

To prevent free radical damage, the body has a defense system of antioxidants. Antioxidants are molecules that can safely interact with free radicals and terminate the chain reaction before vital molecules are damaged. Although there are several enzyme systems within the body that scavenge free radicals, the principal antioxidants are:

glutathione, SOD (superoxide dismutase), beta carotene, vitamin E, vitamin C, CoQ10, melatonin, and alpha lipoic acid.

According to the theory of oxidative stress, free radicals run rampant, wreaking havoc throughout the body. In the case of type 1 diabetes, beta cells in the pancreas are damaged or completely destroyed, thereby negatively impacting their ability to produce insulin. In the case of type 2 diabetes, cell membranes are damaged, leading to a breakdown in intercellular signaling (the pathways responsible for signaling between cells). And if that weren't bad enough, free radicals deplete our body's reserve of antioxidants, further contributing to the problem.

This is why it is so important to lower oxidative stress with better diet, more exercise, and improved lifestyle. It's also critical to take antioxidant supplements to neutralize the excess free radicals. There is still a lot to learn about what causes diabetes, but we do know that our bodies may begin to malfunction five to seven years before we are diagnosed. For this reason, researchers believe that nearly 30–50 percent of those with diabetes don't know they have it (http://www.webmd.com/diabetes/news/20040426/diabetes-rates-worldwide).

In order to treat this illness and eventually reverse it, we need to attack the source of the illness, not put a Band-Aid on it by using prescription medication. I am not denouncing prescription medication; at the onset of this disease, prescription medication is necessary to help the body cope. But as time goes on, to reverse this disease the focus should be on the source of the problem. In order to reverse this disease, it is necessary to understand the role of the pancreas. Understanding how the pancreas works will better equip you with the tools to get this organ healthy.

The Pancreas

Below is a picture of the pancreas and its location with respect to other organs. The pancreas is located in the abdominal cavity (conical-shaped organ shown in picture) behind the stomach at the bend of the duodenum.

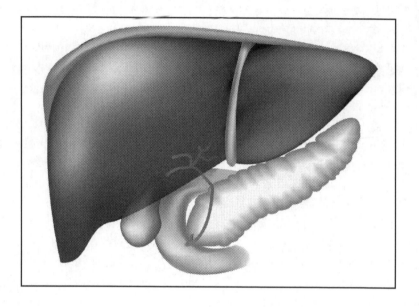

The pancreas has two functional components. The first part is the gastrointestinal tract known as the *exocrine system*, which is responsible for digesting and processing food. The second part is called the *endocrine system*, which secretes the enzyme insulin and also glucagon. Both glucagon and insulin control the level of glucose in the bloodstream. These hormones maintain the balance of sugar in the body and are critical for the proper functioning of the endocrine system.

When the pancreas stop producing insulin, produces too little, or the body does not recognize the insulin, then type 1 or type 2 diabetes set in. How do you know if you have diabetes? The answer is often times *you do not know.* As mentioned earlier in this text, at the time of printing it was estimated that over seven million people in the United States are diabetic and do not know it. People with type 2 diabetes do not always shows symptoms. In my case, the symptoms were all over the place: frequent urination, dizzy spells, weight loss, and you name it; the disease hit me pretty hard. People who develop type 1 diabetes will have a sudden onset of symptoms requiring hospitalization.

Following are some common symptoms of diabetes. Please note that experiencing one or more of these symptoms does not necessarily signal diabetes, but if you have one or more of them, then please see your doctor as soon as possible.

- ✓ increased urination, sometimes as often as every half an hour

- ✓ slow healing wounds

- ✓ thirst, which can be quite excessive

- ✓ blurry vision

- ✓ significant weight loss

- ✓ nausea

- ✓ vomiting

- ✓ itching skin, especially in the groin area

- ✓ extreme fatigue

- ✓ irritability

- ✓ tingling or numbness in the hands or feet

Some of the symptoms for diabetes seem harmless, and as a result many people delay getting medical help. If you experience one or more of these symptoms, please see your doctor who can easily diagnose the condition and start immediate medical treatment. Remember, the sooner a diagnosis is made and treatment is started, the quicker the disease can be brought under control and you can start on your way to reversal.

CHAPTER 3

Risk Factors Associated with Diabetes

- **SEDENTARY LIFESTYLE**

By now we should all know that sitting in front of the television for hours is bad for your health. A number of studies have linked sedentary lifestyle (sitting or resting a lot with very little exercise) with type 2 diabetes, heart disease, and premature mortality. This lifestyle puts one at risk both for becoming obese and for all the other issues that come with being overweight, such as heart disease, diabetes, and hypertension, just to name a few (http://www.webmd. com/fitness-exercise/features/do-you-have-sitting-disease). My advice is to get up from in front of the TV and make sure you exercise at least thirty minutes per day. Once again, I must stress that rigorous exercise is not recommended; instead do moderate exercise such as walking, bowling, golf, gardening, and similar types of exercises. A study conducted by Duke University Medical Center shows that moderate exercise "dramatically lowered" triglycerides levels.

• **GENETICS AND FAMILY HISTORY**

Research shows that genetics plays a role in developing diabetes. Genetics is the study of how parents pass on certain genes to their offspring. People who have family members with type 2 diabetes are at a greater risk for developing it themselves, but environmental factors also play a big role in developing this disease (http://www.diabetes.org/diabetes-basics/genetics-of-diabetes.html). Also, looking at the prevalence of the disease with regard to race reveals that African Americans, Hispanic Americans, and Native Americans have a higher than normal rate of type 2 diabetes.

It is very important to know that having a genetic disposition toward diabetes does not guarantee one will get the disease. In my case, I don't know of any relatives who have the disease. The key words are *I do not know*, because it is possible that others had or currently have the disease and I am not aware of it. It is this type of complacency on my part that got me in trouble. Prior to being diagnosed with the disease, whenever I heard the term *diabetes* I was of the impression that this did not apply to me. Because of this complacency, I did not pay close attention to my eating habits—in particular, my consumption of sugar. I eventually overworked my pancreas, and it got weak and eventually could not cope.

• **INCREASED AGE**

It is no secret that the older you are, the more susceptible you are to diseases. The older we get, the greater the risk of developing diabetes. Sugar metabolism slows down, and that is one reason we tend to gain weight as we age, especially around the belly area. The pancreas also ages right along with your body, and it becomes less efficient in enzyme production and the distribution of insulin. Remember, enzymes in the body are very important for many chemical processes. If you are forty-five or older, it is time to pay closer attention to your eating habits and your general physical health in order to help prevent diseases such as diabetes—although the sooner we all start practicing good eating habits, the better our overall health will be.

• HIGH BLOOD PRESSURE AND CHOLESTEROL

High blood pressure and high cholesterol have been linked to many diseases, including type 2 diabetes. These are major risk factors that must be controlled. High blood pressure and cholesterol wreak havoc on your heart vessels and are the leading causes of metabolic syndrome (previously mentioned), which includes obesity, fatty liver, and several cancers. Having metabolic syndrome increases your risk of heart disease, diabetes, and stroke. If your HDL is 35 mg/dL or lower or your triglyceride levels are over 150 mg/dL, you are at greater risk for heart attacks and strokes. You want to aim for a triglyceride level that is less than 150 mg/dL.

CHAPTER 4

Diabetes Complications

There are many complications associated with diabetes. Therefore, it is absolutely important to keep this disease under control and work toward ridding oneself of this disease. Some of the complications associated with this disease are as follows:

• **KIDNEY FAILURE**

The function of the kidney is to store waste products from digested protein we eat. The waste product is filtered out and becomes part of the urine. Diabetes can damage the kidneys if they filter too much blood, causing them to be overworked. An overworked kidney can become diseased, and this disease can progress to where the kidney loses its filtering ability, resulting in end-stage renal disease. At this stage, waste products gradually build up in the blood, requiring the person to have dialysis or a kidney transplant (http://www. diabetes.org/living-with-diabetes/complications/kidney-disease-nephropathy.html).

- ## VISION PROBLEMS (RETINOPATHY, WHICH CAN LEAD TO BLINDNESS)

Diabetic retinopathy is the most common disease of the eye that is due to diabetes. High blood sugar—and consequently blood sugar spikes—causes retinopathy, which is deterioration of the eye's retina due to diabetes. Diabetic retinopathy has four stages:

1. *Mild nonproliferative retinopathy*: This is the early stage of the disease. At this stage microaneurysms occur. These are tiny swellings in the retina's blood vessels.

2. *Moderate nonproliferative retinopathy*: At this stage, as the disease becomes progressively worse, a number of blood vessels become clogged.

3. *Severe nonproliferative retinopathy*: At this stage, the disease is much more progressive, resulting in more blockages. This leads to deprivation of blood to many areas of the retina.

4. *Proliferative retinopathy*: At this stage, since too many blood vessels are clogged, the retina sends out a signal for nourishment, resulting in the growth of new blood vessels. The danger with creating these new blood vessels is that they are weak and more susceptible to rupture. If rupture occurs, blood is leaked. This leakage can cause severe vision loss and even blindness (http://www.webmd.com/diabetes/eye-health-diabetic-retinopathy).

- ## FOOT COMPLICATIONS

Foot complications are one of the side effects for people with diabetes. If diabetes is not adequately controlled, it can result in nerve damage that can eventually lead to gangrene. Other conditions to be aware of if you have diabetes are as follows:

✓ *Ulcers and calluses:* Ulcers and calluses are common with people who have diabetes. If calluses are not treated and they get very thick, you are at risk for these calluses becoming ulcers. If neglected, ulcers can become infected and even lead to loss of limb.

✓ *Athlete's foot*: This is a common infection caused by a fungus affecting the skin between the toes and is quite common with people with diabetes. As with any open wound or cut, diabetics must be careful to treat this promptly and not risk complications. This condition is treated with antifungal medications such as creams, powders, and ointments.

• HEARING LOSS

According to the National Institute of Health (NIH), hearing loss is twice as common in people with diabetes as it is in those who don't have the disease. This trend is also common with prediabetics. "The 79 million adults thought to have pre-diabetes, the rate of hearing loss are 30% higher than in those with normal blood sugar." (http://www.nidcd.nih.gov/news/releases/08/Pages/06_18_08.aspx).

• ORAL HEALTH (GUM DISEASE)

People with diabetes are more susceptible to bacterial infection; therefore, there is decreased ability to fight germs that invade the gums. When you have gum disease, this results in a buildup of plaque. However, there are many ways you can protect your gums if you have diabetes. Fortunately, frequent brushing, flossing, and regular trips to your dentist can help improve your oral health.

• NERVE DAMAGE (NEUROPATHY)

Neuropathy is a nerve condition often seen in the hands and or feet. This can be caused by a number of factors, but often it is caused by diabetic condition. Poor circulation can cause the nerves to become damaged over time. Damaged nerves may prevent the feeling of heat, cold, and pain, which may lead to serious complications, such as gangrene if there is a cut. Good blood sugar control is a *must* to prevent this condition from developing or progressing.

- **PERIPHERAL ARTERIAL DISEASE**

Many people with peripheral arterial disease (PAD) don't have symptoms. If you do have symptoms, it may be an aching pain in your thigh, in your buttocks, or in your calf. This disease occurs when blood vessels in the legs are narrowed or blocked by fatty deposits. As a result of this blockage, the blood flow to your feet and legs decreases. PAD increases the risk for stroke and heart attack.

- **STROKE**

If you have diabetes, you are at a greater risk for stroke; I'm sorry to be blunt, but that is a fact. Many studies have provided data to show that diabetics are at a greater risk for stroke than nondiabetics. The overall risk of cardiovascular disease is almost three times higher in both men and women with diabetes than for people without the disease. You can lower your risk for stroke by monitoring blood sugar closely on a daily basis and keeping your blood sugar, cholesterol, and blood pressure under control.

- **ALZHEIMER'S DISEASE**

Research has shown that there is a connection between type 2 diabetes and Alzheimer's disease, although there is still some work to be done to fully understand the connection. Research indicates that the connection between the two diseases may be due to blood vessel damage in the brain. Diabetes has been known to damage blood vessels throughout the body, and it is thought that the blood vessel demise in the brain may lead to mild cognitive impairment (MCI), which is linked to Alzheimer's disease. Again, keeping your blood sugar under control can reduce the risk of getting this disease (http://www.mayoclinic.org/diseases-conditions/diabetes/basics/complications/con-20033091).

CHAPTER 5

Taking Charge of Blood Glucose

Before we address lifestyle changes, dietary changes, and ultimately ridding yourself of the disease, once again I want to stress the importance of regular doctor visits. You should also find out if there are any hospitals or other health care facilities in your area that offer diabetes education classes. Remember, understanding as much as possible about this disease will be the key to ridding yourself of it. Your doctor should at a minimum recommend the following tests:

- **LIPID TESTS**

This test measures triglyceride levels and cholesterol. You will want to see results of LDL (bad cholesterol) below 100 mg/dL and your HDL (good cholesterol) above 40 mg/dL, with total overall cholesterol below 200 mg/dL. For the triglycerides, you want to see levels below 150 mg/dL. Levels above 200 mg/dL are considered high and raise the risk for coronary artery disease.

- **HBA1C TESTS**

An HbA1c test, often referred to as simply A1c, will provide you and your doctor information about how well your diabetes has been managed for the previous three months. As mentioned before in the introduction, A1c measures the glucose levels in the bloodstream over a period of generally six to twelve weeks. Glucose sticks to the protein in our red blood cells that carry oxygen. The level of glucose that remains in the bloodstream indicates how well the disease is managed; the less glucose that remains in the bloodstream, the lower the A1c reading. Normal levels for A1c are 4–6 percent. Human red blood cells typically do not live for more than three months, and this test is a good indicator of blood sugar control (http://www.mayoclinic.org/tests-procedures/a1c-test/basics/definition/prc-20012585).

- **C-REACTIVE PROTEIN**

The C-reactive protein test is used to screen for heart disease. Inflammation in the bloodstream has been identified as a leading cause of cardiovascular problems. This test measures the level of inflammation in the bloodstream. Good results are in the range of 1–3 mg/dL, but you should strive to have it at the 1 mg/dL level or less.

- **EYE EXAM**

In addition to visiting your primary care physician, you should go to an ophthalmologist or optometrist. The purpose of this visit is to catch as early as possible any damage to your retina as a result of high blood sugar. Blood vessels in the retina can become damaged.

This condition is known as retinopathy, discussed previously. Your eye doctor will perform a dilated eye exam, in which the pupils are widened with eye drops, to check for signs of diabetic retinopathy.

- **FOOT EXAM**

Individuals who have been diagnosed with diabetes should get a foot exam annually. This exam will identify major issues of the foot that can be caused by high glucose levels over time. According to the American Diabetes Association, the examination should include assessment of protective sensation, foot structure and biomechanics, vascular status, and skin integrity. If you have one or more high-risk foot conditions, you should be evaluated more frequently for the development of additional risk factors. People with neuropathy should have a visual inspection of their feet at every visit with a health care professional.

Foot ulcers and amputations can result in both emotional and physical costs, and they are major causes of disability and morbidity. Early recognition and management of independent risk factors for ulcers and amputations can prevent or delay the onset of adverse outcomes. As reported on the American Diabetes Association website, the recommendations are based on the technical review of care for the nonulcerated foot in diabetes (*Mayfield, J. A. et al.* "Preventive Foot Care in People with Diabetes." *Diabetes Care 21* (1998): 2161–2177).

- **MEASURING BLOOD SUGAR**

You should typically measure blood sugar first thing in the morning before breakfast. You are looking for levels in the range 70–99 mg/dL, which is considered normal. A range of 100–125 is considered to be prediabetes, and 126 and above will put you in the diabetic range. Your aim is to control your blood sugar so that your fasting glucose level is between 70 mg/dL and 100 mg/dL of blood if you are nondiabetic. Two hours after a meal (postprandial), your blood sugar level should be less than 150 mg/dL. If you are diabetic, the American Diabetes association recommends a fasting glucose range of 70 mg/dL to 130 mg/dL, and two hours after eating it should be less than 180 mg/dL (http://www.diabetes.org/living-with-diabetes/treatment-and-care/blood-glucose-control/checking-your-blood-glucose.html).

It's critical to take your blood sugar reading daily. This disease is silent; you may not have—or you may not recognize—symptoms that tell you your blood sugar is high. Most of the cost of blood sugar test strips and meter is usually covered by insurance or Medicare, assuming you have coverage. Once again, please pay attention to your fasting blood glucose level and your postprandial level. This information is vital to helping you manage diabetes as it enables you to make the necessary adjustments to your diet and medication. There are vast selections of blood sugar monitoring meters to choose from and many popular brands available. Below is a picture of the meter I have been using for some time.

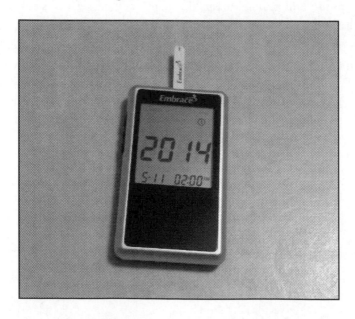

CHAPTER 6

Diet and Exercise

D iet and exercise are two of the most effective ways to control blood sugar and also possibly reverse diabetes. Let us start with diet. When I was first diagnosed, I became very familiar with the term carbohydrates. Bad eating habits are probably the biggest culprit that causes type 2 diabetes; therefore, it is extremely important to limit your sugar intake, especially as you grow older. Over time, sugar builds up in your bloodstream, requiring your pancreas to work harder. The pancreas increases insulin production to cope with increased demands, but eventually the system becomes exhausted and breaks down. With this increased sugar in your system, your body is not able to cope, and the end result is diabetes.

- **DIET**

Foods that contain carbohydrates raise blood glucose. As a diabetic, keeping track of your carbohydrate intake and setting a daily limit can help keep your blood glucose level in your target range. People with diabetes can pretty much eat the same foods as nondiabetics eat, but the trick is it must be done in smaller portions. Although this may be true, there are some foods that are not diabetes-friendly and should be avoided at all costs. Total carbohydrate intake must be monitored. This is where the famous phrase *carbs counting* comes into play (http://www.diabetes.org/food-and-fitness/food/what-can-i-eat/understanding-carbohydrates/).

Let me be extremely clear: diabetics should absolutely learn to do carbohydrates counting, more popularly known as carbs counting. When you go to the supermarket and you pick up a package of biscuits, the label should indicate the total number of grams of carbohydrates in the package, the serving size, and the number of grams of carbs per serving. Please note that one gram is also nicknamed one carb, so the total grams of carbohydrates listed on a food label reading *15 grams of carbohydrates* is commonly referred to as *15 carbs*.

If you have not had diabetes education that teaches you how to count carbs, discuss meal plans, and understand food groups, I strongly recommend that you do. It is recommended that if you are a diabetic you should consume no more than 45 to 60 grams of total carbohydrate at each of your three meals. In addition to reading labels, it is important to understand how many carbs are in foods that are not packaged. Below is a partial list of some common foods containing 15 grams of carbohydrates. Please contact the American Diabetes Association for questions regarding carbohydrate contents of other food types.

For example, there are approximately 15 grams of carbohydrate in the following:

> 1 small piece of fresh fruit (4 oz.)
> 1/2 cup of canned or frozen fruit
> 1 slice of bread (1 oz.) or 1 (6-inch) tortilla
> 1/2 cup of oatmeal

1/3 cup of pasta or rice

4–6 crackers

1/2 English muffin or hamburger bun

1/2 cup of black beans or starchy vegetable

1/4 of a large baked potato (3 oz.)

2/3 cup of plain fat-free yogurt or one sweetened with sugar substitutes

2 small cookies

2-inch square brownie or cake without frosting

1/2 cup ice cream or sherbet

1 tbsp syrup, jam, jelly, sugar, or honey

2 tbsp light syrup

6 chicken nuggets

1/2 cup of casserole

1 cup of soup

1/4 serving of a medium order of french fries

- **EXERCISE**

Exercise is very important for managing type 2 diabetes. Combining diet and exercise can help control type 2 diabetes by

- ✓ improving muscle strength;

- ✓ improving your body's use of insulin;

- ✓ burning excess body fat, helping to decrease and control weight and consequently improve insulin sensitivity;

- ✓ increasing bone density and strength;

- ✓ lowering blood pressure;

- ✓ lowering "bad" LDL cholesterol, which helps to protect against heart disease;

✓ improving blood circulation, consequently reducing your risk of heart disease;

✓ increasing energy level and enhancing work capacity; and

✓ reducing stress, promoting relaxation, and releasing tension and anxiety.

Insulin is normally released from the pancreas when the amount of sugar in the blood increases, such as after eating. Insulin stimulates the liver and muscles to take in excess glucose, which results in lowering the blood sugar level. When exercising, the body needs extra energy or fuel (in the form of glucose) for the exercising muscles. For short bursts of exercise, such as a quick sprint to catch the bus, the muscles and the liver can release stores of glucose for fuel. With continued moderate exercising, however, your muscles take up glucose at almost twenty times the normal rate; this helps lower blood sugar levels.

Intense exercise can have the opposite effect and actually temporarily increase your blood glucose levels right after you stop exercising. This is especially true for many people with type 2 diabetes. The body recognizes intense exercise as a stress and releases stress hormones that tell your body to increase available blood sugar to fuel your muscles; sadly, due to insulin resistance, most of the sugar stays in your bloodstream. If you have diabetes, you may need to check your blood sugar after exercise to see if this happens to you. Please note that it's also possible that your blood sugar is too high for exercise. In some cases, you should hold off exercising if your blood sugar is very high. Ask your doctor to explain under what conditions you should hold off on exercise (http://answers.webmd.com/answers/1194936/how-does-exercise-affect-blood-sugar).

CHAPTER 7

Reversing Diabetes

Modern medicine may not be the most effective treatment for diabetes, especially insulin-resistant diabetes. Medicines that are effective at first gradually lose their potency and leave doctors constantly scrambling to try new combinations, which over time also become less effective. To truly treat this disease and reverse it, we must attack it from the molecular level.

• REIN IN INSULIN

As discussed earlier, insulin is one of the most important hormones in the human body. Our modern lifestyle tends to cause us to overeat. When we do, beta cells in the pancreas go into overproduction mode, producing more insulin to move the glucose molecules into the cells. Over time, the insulin receptor cells become resistant, and the pancreas is not able to keep up with the demands. This leads to type 2 diabetes, high cholesterol, and a host of other diseases. At the molecular level, a person—although not obese—may be genetically predisposed to having abnormal beta cells in the pancreas and as a result develop insulin resistance and diabetes. Treating type 2 diabetes from this perspective is the most effective way to reverse it. (http://7bigspoons.com/rein-insulin/).

- **FIBRINOLYTIC SYSTEMIC ENZYME**

Enzymes are proteins that allow certain chemical reactions in your body to take place much faster than the reactions would occur without them. If you remember high school chemistry, you may recall learning about catalysts and their function to speed up reactions. Enzymes function as catalysts, which means that they speed up the rate at which reactions and metabolic processes occur in the body.

Enzyme therapy (glandular therapy) both with fibrinolytic enzymes or other enzyme types is basically the use of enzymes to treat a specific medical condition or general poor health. At the center of diabetes is an exhausted pancreas that has been worn out due to the excessive demand for insulin. The pancreas is no longer able to keep up with insulin demands and therefore has surrendered. In order to recover from diabetes, we need to give the pancreas time to heal. This is a daunting process, but it can be done and can take from six months to several years; patience is a must. Remember, it took you a long time to develop this chronic condition; a chronic condition requires chronic treatment. The pancreas, in addition to being the insulin factory, has a second role as the body's enzyme factory. Affording the pancreas the opportunity to rest and heal requires taking off the enzymatic load as well (http://www.inflammation-systemicenzymes.com/).

Treating diabetes with fibrinolytic systemic enzymes has been practiced in many countries including Germany, Central Europe, and Japan for over five decades. This treatment has proven to be very effective with no toxicity. Extensive research has been done on treating diabetes with systemic enzymes. You can find peer-reviewed articles online if you search for *systemic enzymes*, and the results will astound you.

The following is a list of some fibronolytic enzymes in use today.

✓ **Lumbrokinase**: This product is fairly new and has found uses in dissolving blood clots and fibrosis (scar tissue), which we all know is caused by inflammation and is a leading cause of peripheral vascular diseases. Diabetes is also one of the leading causes of fibrosis. Lumbrokinase is derived from the earthworm, which for many centuries has been used in the Far East for breaking down fiber. This product should be readily available over the counter (http://nattokinasehearthealth.com/60/what-is-lumbrokinase/).

✓ **Buluoke**: This enzyme is noted for its anticoagulant properties. It is used to treat a myriad of diseases including diabetes, heart disease, malignant tumors, and liver disease. For treatment of acute conditions, the recommended dose is two capsules thirty minutes before meals for 3–4 weeks. For maintenance or prevention, the recommended dosage is one capsule 1–3 times per day, thirty minutes before meals (http://www.biostarorganix.com/boluoke-lumbrokinase/).

✓ **Nattokinase**: This is an all-natural enzyme derived from fermented soy and the bacteria *Bacillus natto*. This enzyme is very effective in treating diseases such as stroke, cardiovascular disease, angina, chronic inflammation and pain, chronic fatigue, tissue oxygen deprivation, hypertension, thrombosis, muscle spasm, and a few others. The recommended dose for therapeutic treatment is 2000 Fibrinolytic Units (FU) bid (twice per day), and for maintenance it is 1000 FU bid (http://www.webmd.com/vitamins-supplements/ingredientmono-1084-nattokinase.

aspx?activeingredientid=1084&activeingredientname =nattokinase).

✓ **Serrapeptase:** This is a proteolytic enzyme that must be consumed in protected tablets or capsules to prevent the stomach acid from destroying it, allowing passage to the intestine where it can be absorbed. Proteolytic enzymes are also known as proteases, and their role is to break down proteins. The effect of serrapeptase is fibrinolytic anti-inflammatory activity, used for sinusitis, sore throat, and ear infection, just to name a few (http://serrapeptase. info/). This enzyme doubles as a pain reducer and is used by physicians throughout Europe and Asia as a pain reliever. The dosage is 10 to 30 mg per day on an empty stomach, preferably divided into three doses.

- **DIABETES AND DIGESTIVE ENZYMES**

In the human body, enzymes play a critical role. Enzymes are manufactured by the body, and they aid in a number of functions, such as digestion, nutrient absorption, maintaining balanced metabolism, providing cellular energy, supporting the brain functions, repairing and healing processes within the body, breaking down toxins, detoxification of blood, and a host of others. One researcher, Dr. Max Wolf, MD, researched enzymes and hormones at Columbia University from the 1930s through the 1960s. The results of Dr. Wolf's researched showed that enzyme production diminishes after the age of 27 (http://www.thewolfeclinic.com/).

Traditionally, humans have been able to supplement their naturally produced enzymes by eating fresh fruits and vegetables, but nowadays preservation and the manner in which foods are prepared are destroying the enzymes these foods contain. The end result is that our bodies become enzyme deficient, and consequently our health suffers. It is essential that we supplement our bodies with enzymes to aid in digestion problems and other deficiencies.

For people with diabetes, pancreatic deterioration affects the production and utilization of insulin. Digestive enzyme supplements may lessen the damage caused by diabetes and also speed up digestion again, and the improved digestion will lead to increased blood sugar control. Type 2 diabetics should pay special attention to *amylase*, a digestive enzyme that helps break down starch into sugar. Amylase is often deficient in people with diabetes, and adding a digestive enzyme supplement containing it could improve blood glucose levels (http://www.livestrong.com/article/370025-what-are-the-functions-of-the-amylase-protease-lipase-digestive-enzymes/).

There are three basic types of enzymes required for our body to sustain life (http://www.gopetsamerica.com/bio/enzyme_types. aspx). Enzyme therapy involves supplementing two of these major enzyme types. The first major enzyme group we will discuss is digestive enzymes, which allow food to be broken down into smaller elements to facilitate digestion. The nutrients are passed into the bloodstream and are eventually moved into the cells by insulin. The second type of enzymes is food enzymes. These are found mostly in raw unfrozen foods and help to digest that particular food. These enzymes digest food in combination with pancreatic enzymes. The more of these available, the fewer pancreatic enzymes your body will need to make. The third type of enzymes is metabolic enzymes. These cannot be supplemented and are used for numerous bodily processes including immune functions, healing, blood cleansing, and so forth. These are the most important enzymes, and they act as the foundation to healing from any medical condition including diabetes. Unfortunately, these cannot be supplemented; they're the ones your body creates.

Pancreatic enzymes aid in digesting food, but they are less important than metabolic enzymes. Proper digestion is vital to metabolic enzymes being used for the right purposes, making pancreatic enzymes just as important. Taking into account the previous paragraph, enzyme therapy would consist mainly of supplementing with pancreatic enzymes, although adding raw, unfrozen foods improves the effectiveness of all supplements significantly. Some popular digestive enzyme supplements on the market are *Pain Power, Cardio Zyme, Super Digesta Zyme, and Pancreatin.*

✓ **Pain Power**

This is an enzyme that is reported to be a good substitute for over-the-counter pharmaceutical medications for pain. Clinical studies show that "serratiopeptidase induces fibrinolytic, anti-inflammatory and antiedemic (prevents swelling and fluid retention) activity in a number of tissues, and its anti-inflammatory effects are superior" (http://www.takebackyourhealth.com/). This is a natural product with no known side effects, and it is non–habit forming. I have used this supplement extensively for over one year with very good results.

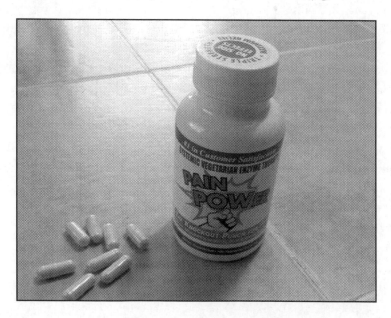

✓ **Cardio Zyme**

Cardio Zyme, otherwise known as Co Enzyme Q-10 or Q-10, is a naturally occurring nutrient in our bodies. Cardio Zyme has been shown to be effective in stimulating the immune system, is a powerful antioxidant, and protects cells from free-radical damage. It can help maintain normal blood pressure and help maintain balanced cholesterol (http://www.takebackyourhealth.com/cardio-zyme. html). We lose Q10 as we age, so taking this supplement will also help combat aging.

✓ **Super Digesta Zyme**

Super Digesta Zyme has been touted as very effective for people with diabetes. We know that the function of digestive enzymes is to break down carbohydrates, proteins, and fats into smaller pieces, so that our bodies can use them more efficiently. Many people with diabetes have some level of pancreatic deterioration; this affects the production of insulin and consequently impairs digestive functions (http://www.takebackyourhealth.com/super-digesta-zyme.html). Super Digesta Zyme lessens the damage done to the pancreas and consequently speeds up digestion.

✓ **Pancreatin**

This enzyme is composed of a mixture of several digestive enzymes that are produced by the exocrine system—namely, amylase, lipase, and protease (http://www.ehow.com/about_5108449_pancreatin-side-effects.html). This supplement is used to treat pancreatitis, inflammation of the pancreas that can lead to digestion problems, making it difficult to digest the food we eat. We also know that—as discussed before—at the heart of diabetes is an inflamed pancreas, making this an essential treatment for diabetes.

• HONEY AND BLOOD SUGAR CONTROL

Many studies have shown that honey has numerous health benefits. One very important benefit of honey is in the control of blood sugar. In many parts of the world, honey is used to promote better blood sugar control. It is absolutely important that the liver is fueled during sleep, and optimal fueling of the liver is paramount to efficient glucose metabolism during sleep and exercise. Raw unheated honey is best; not only does unheated honey provide a surplus of each kind of digestive enzyme, but also it contains an insulin-like factor that has the ability to replace insulin in the body. This benefits the pancreas by relieving both enzymatic and insulin-related duties (http://www.bee-pollen-buzz.com/raw-honey-for-diabetes.html).

After I first learned about the benefits of raw honey I was aggressively downing a few tablespoons at a time; the end result was spiked blood sugar. When I modified the way I consumed it by diluting it in a glass of water, the blood sugar spikes went away. My recommendation is to dilute one tablespoon of raw honey in eight ounces of water, and take it twice per day. Other food sources of enzymes include tropical fruits (especially in unripe form) and fresh vegetable juices, although no other food stacks up to honey.

• SUPPLEMENTS/HERBS

Herbs have been used to treat diabetes for many years. Recent scientific investigation has shown that a host of herbal preparations have been effective in controlling blood sugar. Please note that if you already take oral medication for this disease, you should talk to your doctor regarding your decision to take supplements in lieu of—or in addition to—prescribed medication.

✓ Pterocarpus Marsupium (Indian Kino, Malabar Kino, Pitasara, Venga)

This tree is the source of the Kino of the European pharmacopeias. The gum resin looks like dried blood (Dragon's blood) and is much used in Indian medicine. This herb has a long history of use in India as a treatment for diabetes. The flavonoid (-)-epicatechin, extracted from the bark of this plant, has been shown to prevent alloxan-induced beta cell damage in rats (http://www.idb.hr/diabetologia/09no2-3.pdf).

Both epicatechin and a crude alcohol extract of Pterocarpus marsupium have actually been shown to regenerate functional pancreatic beta cells. No other drug or natural agent has been shown to generate this activity. (The results of this study can be found in "Indian Herbs and Herbal Drugs Used for the Treatment of Diabetes" in *Journal Clinical Biochemistry and Nutrition*, 2007 May 40(3): 163–173.)

✓ Gymnema Sylvestre (Gurmar, Meshasringi, Cherukurinja)

Gymnema assists the pancreas in the production of insulin in type 2 diabetes. Gymnema also improves the ability of insulin to lower blood sugar in both type 1 and type 2 diabetes. It decreases cravings for sweets. This herb may be an excellent substitute for oral blood sugar–lowering drugs in type 2 diabetes. Some people take 500 mg per day of gymnema extract (http://www.ncbi.nlm.nih.gov/pubmed/2259217).

✓ Onion and Garlic (Allium Cepa and Allium Sativum)

Onion and garlic have significant blood sugar lowering action. The principal active ingredients are believed to be allyl propyl disulphide (APDS) and diallyl disulphide oxide (allicin), although other constituents such as flavonoids may play a role as well.

Experimental and clinical evidence suggests that APDS lowers glucose levels by competing with insulin for insulin-inactivating sites in the liver. This results in an increase of free insulin. APDS administered in doses of 125 mg/kg to fasting humans was found to cause a marked fall in blood glucose levels and an increase in serum insulin. Allicin doses of 100 mg/kg produced a similar effect (http://holisticonline.com/remedies/diabetes/diabetes herbs.htm).

Onion extract was found to reduce blood sugar levels during oral and intravenous glucose tolerance tests. The effect improved as the dosage was increased; however, beneficial effects were observed even for low levels around 25 g. The beneficial effects of onion extract were similar for both raw and boiled onion extracts. Onions help increase insulin sensitivity and also help prevent the destruction of insulin.

Allium sativum, otherwise known as garlic, is a putrid pungent herb which is a member of the onion family; it has been shown to have many medical benefits, including lowering cholesterol. It is important for people with diabetes to have cholesterol levels in the acceptable range to avoid complications such as heart disease and stroke. Garlic can be taken raw or in supplements. If you decide to take it raw, it is recommended that you consume two cloves per day. If you decide to take garlic in the supplement form, consume tablets that are equivalent to two cloves of garlic. To calculate how much is needed, look at the allin content on the label. One clove equals 24–56 mg of allin (http://www.webmd.com/cholesterol-management/guide/diseases-linked-high-cholesterol).

The additional benefit of garlic and onions is their cardiovascular effects. They are found to lower lipid levels and inhibit platelet aggregation, and they are also antihypertensive. So, liberal use of onion and garlic are recommended for diabetic patients.

✓ Fenugreek (Trigonella Foenum-Graecum)

Experimental and clinical studies have demonstrated the antidiabetic properties of fenugreek seeds. The active ingredient responsible for the antidiabetic properties of fenugreek is in the defatted portion of the seed that contains the alkaloid trogonelline, nicotinic acid, and coumarin. Fenugreek helps raise the number of insulin receptors in the red blood cells. The recommended dosage is a total of 10 to 15 g one time per day with a meal (http://diabeteshealth.com/read/2005/01/01/4193/fenugreek/).

✓ Blueberry Leaves (Vaccinium Myrtillus)

A decoction of the leaves of the blueberry has a long history of folk use in the treatment of diabetes. The compound myrtillin (an anthocyanoside) is apparently the most active ingredient. Upon injection, it is somewhat weaker than insulin, but is less toxic, even at fifty times the 1 g per day therapeutic dose. A single dose can produce beneficial effects lasting several weeks.

Blueberry anthocyanosides also increase capillary integrity, inhibit free-radical damage, and improve the tone of the vascular system. In Europe, it is used as an antihemorrhagic agent in the treatment of eye diseases, including diabetic retinopathy.

✓ Asian Ginseng

Asian ginseng is commonly used in traditional Chinese medicine to treat diabetes. It has been shown to enhance the release of insulin from the pancreas and to increase the number of insulin receptors. It also has a direct blood sugar-lowering effect.

A recent study found that 200 mg of ginseng extract per day improved blood sugar control as well as energy levels in type 2 diabetes (NIDDM) (http://www.naturaleyecare.com/health-conditions/diabetes-mellitus/).

✓ Bilberry

If you are a diabetic and are more prone to hyperglycemia (high blood sugar levels), you may want to use bilberry as a viable option for high blood sugar control. Bilberry is also touted as very effective in improving blood circulation to the extremities (hands and feet). However, bilberry can lower blood sugar to dangerous levels and may interact with some medications, so please consult your doctor before using it. Bilberry may also lower the risk of some diabetic complications, such as diabetic cataracts and retinopathy (http://www.naturalalternativeremedy.com/bilberry-benefits-and-side-effects/).

✓ Stevia

Stevia has been reported as one of the best sugar substitutes for diabetics. Early reports suggested that stevia might have beneficial effects on glucose tolerance (and therefore potentially help with diabetes), although not all reports have confirmed this (http://healthyeating.sfgate.com/can-diabetics-use-stevia-5868.html). All things considered, if stevia did not have direct antidiabetic effects, its use as a sweetener could help diabetic patients reduce intake of sugars. I have used a derivative of the stevia plant in the form of stevia extract, erythritol, and natural flavors marketed under the name Truvia for all my sweetening needs, and this has been my sugar replacement for many years, with no side effects.

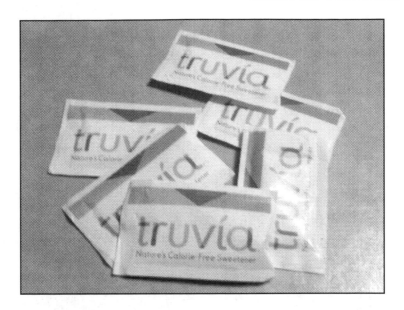

✓ **Ginkgo Biloba**

Ginkgo biloba can help lower blood sugar by stimulating the pancreas to produce more insulin. Studies have shown that in addition to lowering blood sugar, gingko biloba can reduce the damage caused by free radicals and may prove useful for the prevention and treatment of early-stage diabetic neuropathy. Among the other antidiabetic properties is the ability to fight the buildup of plaque in the arteries; it therefore may reduce the risk of heart attack and strokes. Scientific studies have shown that gingko biloba can improve blood circulation by opening up blood vessels and ultimately improve circulation (http://umm.edu/health/medical/altmed/herb/ginkgo-biloba). Again this is very important for people with diabetes who are prone to developing foot problems (neuropathy) due to poor circulation.

✓ **Chia Seeds**

Chia is a flowering plant indigenous to Central America. The seeds of this plant were a staple of the ancient Mayans and Aztecs.

Chia seeds are very rich in fiber and protein but low in fats and carbohydrates, and they can absorb water many times their weight. Chia seeds control blood sugar by slowing down the conversion of carbohydrates to sugar, and they also control insulin resistance. They can be added to your favorite beverage, mixed with water, or consumed raw. Chia seeds are filling, so eating them helps reduce craving—making them an excellent way to help lose weight. They are available in local grocery stores, pharmacies, and specialty food stores.

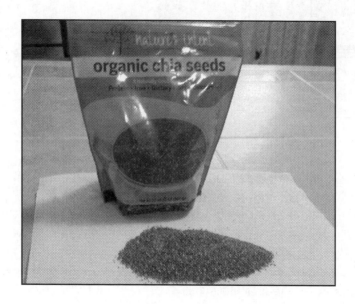

✓ **Eugenia Jambolana**

Eugenia jambolana has been noted for its hypoglycemic (lowering blood sugar) activity. The seeds, the leaves, or the fruits of this plant are effective in lowering blood sugar, but results of studies have shown that the fruit is the most effective. This plant grows in many countries in the world but is native to Bangladesh, Sri Lanka, Philippines, and Pakistan. An extract of the fruit is available in powdered form (http://healthyeating.sfgate.com/).

✓ Ocimum Sanctum (Holy Basil)

This herb is quite popular in India where it is considered to be sacred and is found planted around temples for religious purposes. The plant has been used extensively for medicinal purposes to treat type 2 diabetes, liver ailments, and kidney conditions. In a small controlled-trial diabetes study of forty people with type 2 diabetes, subjects were taken off their diabetes medications seven days before the start of the study. The diabetic patients were then given holy basil leaves as a replacement for their diabetes medication for five days. Twenty participants were given the powdered form of holy basil leaf, and the other twenty were given a placebo for four weeks.

The results showed that for the first group there was a decline in the average fasting glucose from 134.5 mg/dl to 99.7 mg/dl after four weeks of treatment with holy basil. For subjects in the placebo group, their blood glucose increased from 99.7 mg/dl to 115.6 mg/dl (http://diabeteshealth.com/read/2005/09/01/4349/holy-basil-ocimum-sanctum/).

✓ Phyllanthus Amarus

This herb is also commonly known as black catnip, gale of the wind, and stonebreaker—among other names. This is a common herb found in Surinam, and it is used extensively to treat kidney, liver, and gall bladder functions. It is also used for antibacterial and hypoglycemic applications, as well as for treatment of inflammation of the appendix, for diabetes, and also prostate problems (http://www.tropilab.com/black-cat.html).

✓ Trigonella Foenum Graecum

Trigonella foenum graecum is a medicinal plant commonly found in India and North Africa (http://www.herbal-information.com/

fenugreek-trigonella-foenum-graecum/). It has been reported to be very effective for controlling blood sugar. Studies have shown that this herb helps increase the number of insulin receptors, thereby lowering blood glucose. When combined with bitter melon, diabetic patients reported significantly reduced fasting and postprandial glucose levels.

✓ Withania Somnifera

This herb is also commonly known as Ashwagandha and is used widely all over the world for medicinal purposes, especially in India. Studies have shown this to be a powerful antioxidant that can also reduce blood sugar and cholesterol. A study conducted in type 2 diabetic rats that were fed 200 to 400 mg/kg of Withania somnifera once per day for five weeks showed significant improvement in their blood glucose levels (http://www.cpmedical.net/articles/ashwagandha-withania-somnifera-improves-glucose-tolerance-in-rodents). Several studies have also shown that Withania somnifera has anti-inflammatory, antitumor, antistress, antioxidant, immune enhancing and mind-boosting properties.

✓ Cinnamon

Although cinnamon is considered by many to be a natural product for lowering blood sugar, there is conflicting information regarding whether it actually does. A 2008 review published in the journal *Diabetes Care* found no benefits to diabetics using cinnamon. However, a later study conducted in 2010 and published in the journal *Diabetic Medicine* showed lower blood sugar levels in the group that took two grams of cinnamon per day for twelve weeks. Regardless of how inconclusive the studies are, there is evidence that foods seasoned with cinnamon do lower the blood sugar response.

✓ Barberry—One of the Mildest and Best Liver Tonics Known

Barberry has shown to be a very effective medicinal plant. This herb is traditionally used for liver problems and promotes the flow of bile. Recent studies have shown that this herb has a significant inhibiting effect on diabetes. It stimulates the immune system, activates macrophages (big eaters), and is considered a scavenger of free radicals; it consequently may inhibit the progression of diabetes (http://www.itmonline.org/arts/berberine.htm).

✓ Curcumin

Curcumin is a major component of the turmeric plant. This agent has significant health benefits for diseases such as fatty liver disease, Alzheimer's, tendinitis, and Rift Valley Fever virus. This herb is a member of the ginger family, and according to a study from researchers at Harbin Medical University and the Chinese Center for Disease Control and Prevention, curcumin reduces levels of free fatty acids (FFAs) in patients with type 2 diabetes. Why is reducing free fatty acids important? The answer is simple; free fatty acids are a main culprit in the development of insulin resistance. Curcumin is an excellent anti-inflammatory that acts by suppressing the inflammatory cytokines produced by the immune cells in the fatty tissue that cause heart damage and also damage to the insulin-producing pancreatic islands.

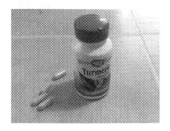

✓ **Tea—Green and Black**

The results of an animal study have shown that green tea and black tea are both helpful in controlling high blood sugar in rats. The results of the study also show that green and black tea may prevent diabetic animals from developing cataracts. The findings appear in the May 4, 2005, issue of the *Journal of Agricultural and Food Chemistry.* "Black and green tea represent a potentially inexpensive, nontoxic, and, in fact, pleasurable [blood-sugar-lowering] agent," the researchers write. "Tea may be a simple, inexpensive means of preventing or retarding human diabetes and the ensuing complications."

In the study, researchers gave green and black tea to diabetic rats for three months. They found both kinds of tea inhibited diabetic cataracts. The teas also lowered blood sugar levels. To get the same dose of tea given to the rats, a 143-pound person would have to drink 4.5 8-ounce cups of tea every day. The researchers recommend that tea—black and green—should be studied for an antidiabetes effect in humans. Dosage: tincture, 10–30 drops; standard decoction or 3–9 g (http://www.webmd.com/diabetes/news/20050420/black-tea-green-tea-good-for-diabetes).

✓ **Bitter Melon (Momordica Charantia)**

One of the most amazing natural substances touted as a possible cure for diabetes is bitter melon, also known as bitter gourd or Momordica charantia. According to Diabtesguide.com, bitter melon (which is classified as a vegetable) is grown in many tropical countries: the Philippines, India, China, and Malaysia. This vegetable has been recognized as a very good treatment for diabetes, and in some cases (as mentioned before) has been said to be a possible cure for this disease. The compound responsible for the hypoglycemic property is *charntin.* As you can see from the picture, this vegetable has a conical shape and measures approximately 10 to 20 centimeters in length.

Some of the other benefits that have been mentioned are in the treatment of cholera, blood disorders, alcoholism, and HIV http://www.bitter-gourd.org/).

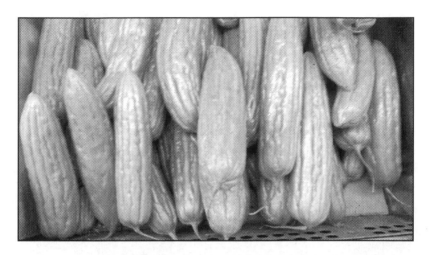

So how does bitter melon achieve this? The results of scientific research show that bitter melon controls blood sugar by preventing the buildup of glucose in the bloodstream. It acts as a mediator between the body cells and insulin and opens up the cells (breaking down the barriers), making the cells more receptive to insulin.

The recommended dose is five to ten grams of the juice with or without water three times a day, for two to three months. The oral administration of 50–100 ml (1.7–3.4 oz) of the juice has shown good results in clinical trials. However this dose may be adjusted based on your blood sugar levels and whether or not you take conventional drugs for diabetes.

Bitter melon is also used to treat liver failure, one of the complications of diabetes. Liver failure is a life-threatening condition that demands immediate medical care. If detected early, liver failure can often be treated and its effects reversed. Several traditional therapies use the extract of bitter melon to treat liver conditions successfully. However, consult with a physician before using alternative therapies for any medical condition. Studies have also shown that bitter melon is not only valuable in controlling blood glucose, but also has antioxidant potential to protect vital organs, such as the liver, against damage caused by diabetes-induced oxidative stress. Another study published in the *Journal of Nutrition* in April 2003 found that bitter melon extract improved insulin resistance and also reduced high blood sugar in laboratory animals in the test.

How does it work? Using extractions from bitter melon (cucurbitane triterpenoids), researchers were able to show that in mice, bitter melon could stimulate parts of the body's glucose metabolism system. When bitter melon extract was present, the glucose receptor in the fat and muscle cells moved toward the surfaces of the cells. This then allowed for the removal of sugar from the blood stream (much like insulin does) (http://tcmnutra.com/bitter-melon-blood-sugar/).

Caution: Excessively high doses of bitter melon juice can cause abdominal pain and diarrhea. Small children or anyone with hypoglycemia should not take bitter melon, since this herb can theoretically trigger or worsen low blood sugar (hypoglycemia). Furthermore, diabetics taking hypoglycemic drugs (such as chlorpropamide, glyburide, or phenformin) or insulin should use bitter melon with caution, as it may potentiate the effectiveness of the drugs, leading to severe hypoglycemia. In the next section, you will be presented with a step-by-step approach to managing your blood sugar. I have had very good results with some of these techniques.

CHAPTER 8

Step-by-Step Method

In the previous chapters I have provided a lot of information about diabetes. Now let us see what you can do to rein in this disease if you are one of the approximately 350 million afflicted by it.

I have spoken about the role of diet in causing this disease, and consequently diet plays an important role in reversing it. Note I use the term *reversing* versus *cure*. If you are serious about controlling the effects of type 2 diabetes, you can live a normal life—and even be healthier than people who do not have this disease. At present there is no cure, although there is promising research that may lead to a cure in the future. Pancreatic transplant is currently available for type 1 diabetes patients, especially if the diabetes cannot be controlled with insulin. Also, if there is kidney damage due to uncontrolled diabetes, one option is a combination of pancreatic transplant and kidney transplant. I have no statistics on the success of these transplants, but as you can imagine, there may be complications. Please note that this type of treatment is not recommended for type 2 diabetics.

Doctors see some promise with using stem cells to cure diabetes. Researchers have found that when human embryo stem cells are converted into insulin-producing cells and injected into diabetic mice, the treatment alleviates diabetes in the rodents (http://abcnews. go.com/Health/DiabetesResource/story?id=4318544&page=1). Although this study took place several years ago, the research continues.

For type 2 diabetics, another breakthrough treatment now in use is the fetal stem cells implant. The cellular building blocks are administered both intravenously (within a vein) and subcutaneously (under the skin), or in some case directly into the pancreas using a catheter. The stem cells then travel through the body and attempt to repair and restore damaged cells. Reversing diabetes means getting it under control so you become less dependent on prescription medication. As mentioned earlier, before you embark on any treatments called out in this text, please consult your physician or another health care specialist, such as your dietician.

- **STEP 1: CHANGE YOUR DIET**

One of the most important steps in controlling diabetes, both type 1 and type 2, is diet. Research has shown that poor diet is one of the major contributing factors for diabetes. Processed foods, overcooked foods, and overconsumption of sugar/carbohydrates tax the body to the limit and may result in the breakdown of the body—and subsequently, the onset of diabetes.

I recommend a diet rich in fruits (pay attention to the sugar content and limit as needed), vegetables, raw foods, unprocessed foods, and fiber. These foods already have live enzymes (found in all raw and unprocessed foods) to aid in digestion. Since these "live" foods by design have sufficient enzymes to aid in digestion, your body does not have to turn to its reserve to aid in the digestion process.

Whenever you can switch to the organic variety of foods, you will get more nutrients than from foods grown in soil lacking the essential minerals. I have cut out red meat completely from my diet. I will not tell you why because I do not want the beef people coming after me, but please research red meat and diabetes and you will see why. The picture that follows is an example of what my meal looks like nowadays.

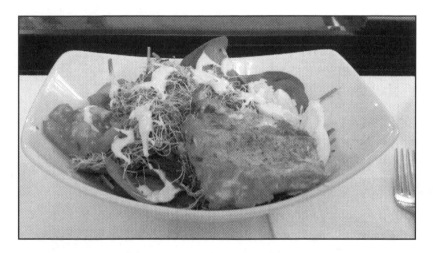

The following is a list of some foods that are safe and some that should be avoided. This is not a complete list, of course, and I advise anyone who has diabetes to consult with his or her nutritionist for dietary advice, as this section is for information only.

Foods that are safer for diabetics:

✓   Good carbohydrates:

This includes whole grains, fruits, and vegetables. Although there is a long list of healthy (complex carbohydrates) for diabetics you should strive to eat only carbohydrates that have a low glycemic index (GI). Glycemic index is the rate at which carbohydrates are absorbed into the bloodstream.

The following is a list of some complex carbohydrates that are diabetic friendly. This list is by no means complete, but it's a starting point:

Whole grain or multigrain foods such as rye bread, whole wheat flour breads and pastas, whole grain cereals, steamed broccoli, broccoli rabe, celery, mixed green salads, mushroom, arugula, cucumber, lettuce, radish, turnip, romaine lettuce, iceberg lettuce, green pepper, red pepper, yellow pepper, okra, cauliflower, cabbage, spinach, green beans, carrots, kale, snap peas, and onions.

Recommended healthy carbohydrates of the fruit variety are:

Watermelon, casaba melon, honeydew melon, strawberries, cantaloupe, avocado, blackberries, grapefruit, oranges, peaches, papayas, cranberries, plums, raspberries, pineapple, nectarines, blueberries, apples, pears, kiwi fruit, cherries, tangerines, mangoes, and persimmons.

✓ Healthy protein:

Unlike carbohydrates, proteins generally have little effect on blood sugar, but there are exceptions. Protein is an essential nutrient for diabetics, however. Recommended sources of protein are chicken, turkey, fish, crab, lobster, shrimp, lamb chop, eggs, and nuts such as walnuts, peanuts, hazelnuts, pecans, almonds, pistachios, cashews, and macadamias.

✓ Foods to avoid:

White rice, white bread, soda, white potatoes, ice cream, cream cheese, cookies, cakes, pies, butter, white flour and white flour products, overripe bananas, canned vegetables, sugar substitutes such as aspartame, and foods containing high fructose corn syrup. Be forewarned that consuming excess amounts of foods (especially meat products, which have a high fat content) leads to a later breakdown of them into fat in the digestive system; this can also spike blood sugar. Studies have also found that the saturated fat in meat can lead to coronary heart disease, yet another danger.

• STEP 2: ADD SUPPLEMENTS TO YOUR DIET

As we age, every organ and system in our bodies also ages. When we are young, our bodies have an optimal supply of endogenous enzymes (originating inside the body), but over time these decline to less than desirable levels that must be supplemented. Here is a brief description and recap of enzymes.

There are two sources of enzymes:

(1)   Exogenous (originating outside the body)

(2)   Endogenous (originating within the body)

These are further broken down into (a) food enzymes found in raw unprocessed foods, (b) digestive enzymes, which help the body digest food, and (c) metabolic enzymes, which are primarily produced and released by the pancreas. When our supply of enzymes declines as our body ages, we become disease-ridden, and then we die.

It is therefore absolutely necessary to restore the supply of enzymes to optimal levels for good health. Over time, one of the most serious threats to enzyme depletion is consuming processed and overcooked foods. By overcooking or processing food, we essentially destroy the enzymes; consequently, when we consume this type of food, the body must turn to the enzyme reserves in our bodies. This eventually leads to depletion, so we must then supplement with exogenous enzymes. There are many brands of enzymes on the market, but I prefer the following:

(a) Pain Power, (b) Cardiozyme, (c) Super Digestazyme, and (d) pancreatin. Again, please discuss with your doctor before taking any enzyme supplements.

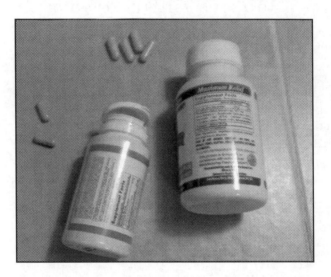

✓ Add vitamin supplements to your diet:

At a minimum, add a supply of the essential vitamins below. Once again, please consult your doctor before you take any supplements. If you are low on vitamin D—which many people are—this is an essential supplement to take. Most of the vitamin D we get is from exposure to sunlight, and unfortunately most of us do not get sufficient sunlight. Vitamin D treats conditions such as diabetes, heart and blood vessel issues, osteoporosis, and a host of other diseases.

Vitamin A Deficiency: Children are particularly susceptible to this deficiency, but it can affect both young and old with serious consequences. Vitamin A deficiency can cause blindness; the outer layer of the eyes can become cloudy, and if left untreated it can lead to complete loss of vision. Vitamin A deficiency can also result in skin problems, whereby the skin becomes dry, rough, and dead looking; it can also make one more susceptible to infectious diseases. Foods rich in vitamin A are carrots, sweet potato, kale, spinach, squash, cantaloupe, and sweet red peppers. Of course this is not an extensive list. Talk to your doctor, and if your vitamin A reserves are low, your doctor may be able to recommend a suitable supplement.

Vitamin B1 Deficiency: Vitamin B1 is essential to give the body the energy required to process carbohydrates. As a diabetic, lacking this vitamin adds complications to a system already struggling to process carbohydrates. Most of us should be able to get sufficient vitamin B1 from the foods we eat, because many packaged foods (such as cereals) have this important vitamin added. Please add this important vitamin to your supplement list if your doctor agrees. Also, please limit alcohol consumption, as this is one of the primary culprits in causing this deficiency.

Vitamin B2 deficiency (like B1) affects your energy, the metabolism of carbohydrates, ketone bodies, fats, and protein in your body. A diet rich in meat, nuts (such as almonds), green leafy vegetables, and whole grains should provide you with sufficient vitamin B2; however, if your doctor is in agreement that you are deficient, the recommended supplement dosage is 1.3 mg per day for women, and 1.7 mg per day for men.

Vitamin C Deficiency: Deficiency of vitamin C is associated with fatigue, chronic pain in joints, mood changes, and weight loss. If you are experiencing these symptoms, however, it may have nothing to do with a lack of vitamin C, so it is important to talk to your doctor first to see whether you suffer from this deficiency. From the diabetic perspective, a lack of this vitamin will affect the way wounds heal. Wounds typically heal more slowly for diabetics, and if you are deficient in vitamin C, they heal even more slowly. Also, a vitamin C deficiency makes you more prone to infections. Foods rich in vitamin C are broccoli, kiwi, oranges, dark green leafy vegetables, yellow peppers, tomatoes, strawberries, and guava. Please consult your doctor and if it is decided that you are lacking vitamin C, adding vitamin C supplements to your diet may be a good idea. In the next section we cover the importance of managing stress in reversing and managing diabetes.

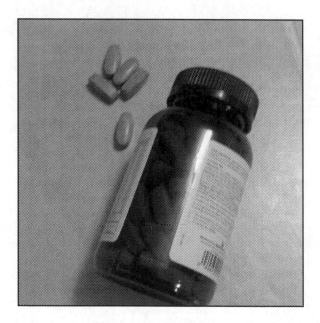

• **STEP 3: STRESS MANAGEMENT**

It has been my observation talking to many people who are diabetic that most do not understand the devastating affect that stress—if not properly managed—can have on diabetics. Some months ago I experienced an event that was very stressful, and I was very surprised that my fasting blood glucose was over 200 mg/dL. It has been quite a long time since I have seen any numbers in that range. I have stuck to my diet and frequently take a number of supplements that I have described in this text, yet none of that was sufficient to counteract the fight-or-flight reaction that stress causes.

The fight–or–flight response is the body's psychological and biological reaction to perceived danger. In preparation for this danger, the liver releases a vast amount of glucose to provide energy to deal with the situation. The longer one remains in that stressful frame of mind, the longer your body will take to resume a balanced state. As you can imagine, frequent stress will negatively affect blood sugar control. Talk to your doctor regarding stress management, and take steps to avoid getting into stressful situations. If you cannot avoid stressful situations, please learn stress management skills to help cope.

• STEP 4: EXERCISE REGULARLY

Regular exercise is one of the best ingredients for health. I cannot stress the importance of exercise enough in maintaining good health, and it also helps the healing process if you have a chronic illness. For diabetes management, it is extremely important that you find time to exercise at least thirty minutes a day for at least five days a week; however seven days would be better. Exercise improves the body's ability to use insulin more effectively by strengthening muscles; this helps the muscles pull the glucose from your bloodstream and into the cells where it is needed. Moderate exercise is preferred; studies have shown that moderate–intensity endurance exercise is more effective than short bursts. Moderate exercise such as walking, bowling, and golf allow the muscles to draw glucose at twenty times the normal rate, thus lowering blood sugar. Short bursts exercise the muscle, and the liver releases glucose for fuel.

How do we define what is moderate versus what is high intensity? If you are doing moderate aerobic exercise, you are exercising at a pace to get your heart rate up and sweat a little, but you should still be able to carry on a conversation. With a more vigorous exercise, you should not be able to carry on a conversation without trying to catch your breath.

- **STEP 5: TEST OFTEN**

One key to effective blood glucose control is to know your numbers. Let's face it; you cannot control your blood glucose if you do not know what it is. Two hours after a meal, you should test your blood glucose to see what is going on. The information you receive will help you adjust diet, adjust exercise schedule, and pretty much paint a picture of where you are in managing your diabetes. *What should be your target?* you may ask. You should always consult your doctor regarding what your target should be. According to The American Diabetes Association, you should be below 180 mg/dL two hours after a meal, but The American Association of Clinical Endocrinologists has set a lower target of below 140 mg/dL.

- **STEP 6: REGULAR DOCTOR VISITS**

Diabetes health management specialists recommend a doctor's visit every three to six months. I would say you should make it every three months. This will allow you and your doctor to see how well your diabetes management is going and to make necessary adjustments in a timely manner. You should also have regular eye exams and foot exams, recommended at least once a year. Some of the things your doctor should check for are: foot infections, calluses, and loss of feeling in your feet. The doctor assesses the loss of feeling in your feet using a special tool that has the feel of a thin blade of grass; this is moved around under your foot bottom to see if you can feel the sensation.

During your regular visits, your doctor should have your results from A1c (hopefully you did the lab test). You should also have your results about triglycerides level and, once per year, a kidney test. For the kidney test, they will be looking for a protein called albumin to see what level you have in your urine. Higher levels could indicate early kidney issues, although other factors unrelated to kidney damage could result in higher than normal albumin in your urine.

CHAPTER 9

Summary

In this text you have been presented with some very valuable information that, if followed, could save your life and let you avoid serious diabetes complications, such as loss of limbs, blindness, kidney failure, heart attacks, and strokes. Diabetes is not very well understood. As with many other chronic diseases, current treatments are designed to treat symptoms rather than cure the condition. This is a disease that will get progressively worse if care is not taken to limit blood sugar spikes or if you don't keep your blood sugar within the recommended blood sugar range (below 140 mg/dL).

The role of diet in controlling diabetes has not been emphasized enough. Control your diet by staying away from foods that could spike your blood sugar. Instead, eat foods that will provide the necessary nutrients for healthy living. The role of vitamin deficiency was also discussed. Vitamin deficiency may have contributed to the onset of diabetes in the first place. Sadly, we do not get sufficient vitamins from the foods we eat for a myriad of reasons. It is therefore necessary to identify which vitamins your body is lacking and take steps to consume the right foods—and, if necessary, add vitamin supplements.

The role of stress was discussed. This is one of the most important areas to control if you are a diabetic. You do not want to get into that fight-or-flight situation that stress creates; your body will pump sugar from its reserves to help you through this impending danger, the way the body sees this threat. This sudden burst of sugar in your bloodstream can create an unhealthy blood sugar spike; therefore, please avoid stressful situations. In the event this not possible, you must learn stress coping skills.

In this text, we introduced the role that enzymes play in your body and the need to eat enzyme-rich foods. Dead food (processed and overcooked) has been credited with causing many of the chronic debilitating illnesses that currently exist today. Enzyme-rich foods such as fruits and vegetables must be a regular part of your diet, and it is always a good idea to go one step further and add enzyme supplements to your diet.

The role of exercise in diabetes control has also been discussed. Exercise provides a number of benefits, such as helping you lose weight, if needed, and helping strengthen your muscles for insulin uptake. Exercise moderately at least thirty to forty-five minutes a day, and you should see the results in your blood sugar levels.

Lastly, the importance of regular doctor visits to monitor your blood sugar control is extremely important. Diabetes can be a silent, deadly disease. The symptoms of high and low blood sugar can be very subtle and could result in these symptoms being ignored. Regular doctor visits—when the necessary laboratory tests results are discussed—will help you and your doctor devise and assess your diabetes management. These visits should be at least every three months so that necessary adjustments can be made in a timely manner.

I hope the information I have presented here has been helpful, and I will continue to research and provide information that I hope will help prevent disastrous consequences due to this debilitating illness.